Healthy Brain, Healthy Gut, Healthy Life

───── ✥✥✥✥ ─────

How Anti-Inflammatory Diet Can Relieve Stress and Anxiety

Candere Publishing Company

regarding its prolonged validity or interim quality. Trademarks that are mentioned are done without written consent and can in no way be considered an endorsement from the trademark holder.

Table of Contents

Introduction

Congratulations on downloading *Healthy Brain, Healthy Gut, Healthy Life: How Anti-Inflammatory Diet Can Relieve Stress and Anxiety* and thank you for doing so.

The following chapters will discuss the anti-inflammation diet and what it can do to help or inhibit physical and mental health. The chapters will discuss the seriousness of depression and anxiety and how inflammation can play a key role in the development of both. They will also explain the difference between acute and chronic inflammation as well as how each interacts with the rest of the body. This book describes what they are and why the body triggers each response. What effect each has on the mind will be discussed as well. It also leads into how nutrition plays a significant role in the body's inflammation. This book will provide background information on Dr. Andrew Weil, the creator of the anti-inflammation diet. The chapters break down the components of the diet and explain each aspect, such as calorie count, guidelines, and meal examples. Also included is a list of anti-inflammation foods and what categories of micronutrients, fats, carbohydrates or proteins, that they fall under. This book also discusses how pro-inflammatory foods can contribute to depression, anxiety, and stress. Additionaly, it provides the breakdown of what is in unhealthy foods that make them so detrimental to the body. There is also a chapter on the connection between intestinal health, hormones, and the brain. It will provide examples of how the microbes that reside in the stomach and mental health seem to be two sides of the same coin, and how repairing one may also repair the other. It also explains the other ways that gut microbes benefit the body, mind, and life of the person from which they reside. After reading this book, you'll have the tools to make the best dietary choices possible, and as a result, you can have the healthiest body and the happiest mind possible!

There are plenty of books on diet and health on the market, thanks again for choosing this one! Every effort was made to ensure it is full of as much useful information as possible, please enjoy!

Chapter 1:
Acute Versus Chronic
Inflammation

How are depression, anxiety, autism, autoimmune diseases, fatigue, hormonal complications, and gastrointestinal bacteria all connected? Well, the answer isn't simple. They are all interwoven in ways that aren't all understood yet, and how changing one affects the others isn't always obvious. No one completely understands the, often, delicate balances and connections within the body. However, one major connection that seems to combine them all together is inflammation. Discussed in this chapter is how inflammation, when at persistent and high levels, can lead to seemingly different types of seemingly unrelated health problems. Explained within this book is a detailed explanation on how inflammation affects the body and mind, and how other centers of the body can be inhibited by overactive, or chronic, inflammation. As the chapters progress, they will explain more about how a body's inflammation can affect hormonal balances within the body, the mental health status a person lives with, and what can be done to reduce these problems by focusing on the inflammation itself. Discussed is how diet, fitness, types of food and chemicals can affect inflammation and what should be done to help fight chronic inflammation before it leads to an incurable disease.

It's nearly 1 PM, five hours later than when you promised yourself you'd get out of bed. However, you're still curled up on the mattress. The curtains are drawn over the window so that the room is as dark as possible, and the covers are pulled up to your chin. In the darkness, your mind spins with responsibilities and chores that need to get done. But try as you might, you just can't force yourself to rise and start your day. The effort from trying to so much as push the blanket off of you leaves the muscles in your fingers straining as you tightly grip the edge that's tucked under your chin. You stare across the room at the wall you know is green. In this light, it looks black. You try to stare hard enough to see the color to distract from the racing thoughts going through your head. The effort of this small act is exhausting, but you fight through it anyway. Your palms begin to sweat as the force of your day presses in on you. The longer you wait, the less time you'll have. The less time you have, the more you panic. The more you panic, the more your body fights you on leaving this bed. Your mind jumps to the important phone call you need to make that day, and your heart beats a little faster from the thought alone. Dancing through your mind is the many ways you could get out of it. You could simply say you forgot until you receive a notice in the mail. You could make up a funeral you had to attend. You could pretend you lost your voice from illness. None of these plans are logical. The call will take ten minutes at most and then the weight of it will leave your mind. So what if you stumble over your words? So what if you forget what you're calling about? It's a complete stranger on the other end of that phone. You try to use this logic to calm yourself down and will your body to relax enough to stand, but you feel so tired and worn out despite how little you've done today. Your mind bounces back and forth between the panic of your responsibilities and wondering why it even matters anymore. The dark creature in the back of your mind eggs you on with promises that none of your friends or family really care about you, and that they wouldn't care if you never showed your face again. That you might as well remain in your pajamas all day until you wither away. You do your best to ignore them. It is now two pm. The day is over half over now. You turn your face into the pillow and drown out the sounds of birds and the carefree chatter of neighbors. You envy them and their ability to easily communicate with others outside where the sun is shining while you have to walk yourself through how to manage to get out of bed. You remind yourself that this is a bad day and that most are usually more manageable than this. It's nearly night time, by the time everything is done. On a good day it could have all been finished and done with before noon, and you would have more time to do something you enjoyed. You remind yourself it doesn't matter because you wouldn't have been able to do those things either. As you go to sleep, you hope tomorrow isn't like today.

This scenario is an example of what some of the harder days can look like through the eyes of someone who suffers from both depression and anxiety. Hopelessness, a lack of motivation, extreme tiredness and fatigue, and the dark thoughts of isolation stem from depression. Depression is a mental disorder that plagues the mind with such thoughts. Someone with major depression will feel a kind of sadness that won't feel like the sharp cut of grief or the sour heaviness of disappointment. It can feel like a combination of bitter loneliness, a sense of despair, a feeling of loss, and a low drive to do what the person normally enjoys doing. Hobbies will be abandoned, work ignored, and friends and loved ones will be avoided. These feelings are often persistent and constant. Signs that someone suffers from depression can include frequent drowsiness and sleeping more often than is normal, irritated at everything and everyone, low drive to take care of themselves or their appearance, forgetfulness, a feeling of numbness throughout the body, and suicidal thoughts or tendencies. Depression is a very real and dangerous mental illness. And yet, because there isn't anything outwardly wrong with the person, it often is disregarded for sadness or laziness. However, an average day to any other person could feel like a tragedy to someone with depression, even though they can't explain why. On good days, the presence of the depressive symptoms are minimal, and the person can go about their day with moderate ease. On these days, motivation, social interaction are doable and can even be enjoyable. However, on harder days, like the one in the scenario, even the smallest responsibility feels like too much.

Anxiety is another mental disorder. It is when a person feels a constant state of unease and panic or feels this in excess. Often a person with anxiety suffers it daily, as social or new tasks can cause distress no matter how minimal. A triggering event, which is different for each person, can set them off or push their anxiety over the edge. This is where anxiety attacks or panic attacks can happen. Panic attacks are often portrayed as the person curling up into the fetal position, hyperventilating, rocking themselves or sometimes screaming. Though these can be signs of a panic attack, it doesn't always look at this. It can be subtle. The person can display signs such as elevated breathing or spacing out at an inappropriate time. They might cry or withdraw into themselves to avoid any more social interaction. When these two are combined, and they often are, the scenario described above is one way it can show. A mixture of panic over what needs to be done, but also a lack of motivation from the depression. On favorable occasions, this can be overcome by sheer force of will or outside aid. On others, however, the mental disorders might win.

Each year, an average of 44,965 suicides occur per year in the United States, and for every successful suicide, there are 25 attempts. Nearly 75% of those successful suicides were by people who suffered from major depression in their days leading up to their deaths. About 6.7% of the United States population suffers from major depression, and around 18.1% suffer from anxiety disorders. That comes to about 16.1 million Americans who suffer depression and 40 million from anxiety in their daily lives. Often a person who lives with one suffers the other as well. These shockingly high numbers have led doctors and scientific researchers to search for cures or aids to lower and even eliminate both the symptoms of both depression and anxiety. Different treatments from psychiatrists, psychologists, and medical doctors exist in different forms such as talk therapy, antidepressants and antianxiety medicines, and eye-movement desensitization and reprocessing or EMDR. Although treatments and medications help alleviate symptoms and make it easier to cope with depression and anxiety, they aren't always enough to completely eliminate the problem itself. Often, medications only treat symptoms of depression and anxiety and provide temporary relief to help make daily life more manageable. They don't actually locate the origin of its source. Like these mental health complications, many medical problems are treated by their symptoms and not the initial source that created them in the first place. However, unless the first ring in the chain of medical complications is removed, they will never go away completely.

But, then, what is the root of the problem? This is a question that many have pondered, and the answer seems to change each time it is asked. Unfortunately, not all depression is alike. Some are obtained from a traumatic event leading to Post-Traumatic Stress Disorder or PTSD. Others can be hereditary. Various therapies are available in the world to cope with the existing disorders, however, because these are temporary aids, the struggle persists. One connection to both that, perhaps, not everyone has made, however, is chronic inflammation. One man, Dr. Andrew Weil, had studied how chronic inflammation affects the body and the mind, and how to lower it by a natural means that has no drawbacks. He found that the best way to do so is to change one thing that could start a chain reaction to better health. Both physically and mentally. By alleviating the root symptom that affects so much of the body and its functions, you can tackle multiple other symptoms as a result. This important change is switching to, and sticking with, the anti-inflammation diet.

Before understanding the anti-inflammation diet, it is important to understand inflammation itself. There are two types of inflammation. One is vital to everyday life and saves it on a daily basis. The other is a serious medical problem that inevitably leads to more and more physical and mental problems the longer it goes on. It can create a chain reaction of problems throughout each system of the body. Because of this, problems will arise within the endocrine system, the cardiovascular system, the neurological system, and mental health. As this inflammation can cause diseases, worsen them, or both, knowing what it is and what can cause it is vital to understanding just how serious of a concern it can be.

When a child is playing at a park and falls, he or she might scrape their knees against the unsanitary gravel beneath the playground equipment. The immune system within the child's body will detect the damage and trigger what is known as an acute inflammatory response to repair it. In a healthy person, the inflammation response will redirect blood flow to the damaged area and surround it with blood. The components of blood are: plasma, white and red blood cells and red blood platelets. Cells that are a part of the body are marked with antigens that let the white blood cells know they are not invaders. If a foreign microorganism, such as a virus or bacteria, enters the body through an injury such as the child's scraped knees, the white blood cells will attack and ingest them to prevent the invaders from duplicating and invading the body. During this time, the injured area will swell slightly due to the secreted fluids from the white blood cells and the plasma build up. The skin cells around the wound will become warm to the touch as the white cells attack the intrusion, much like a healthy fever during a cold or flu. The redirected blood is thickened with extra red platelets that pool together in the damaged area and close off the opening to the body. This will form a scab, which acts as a temporary cap to the injury until the skin can heal itself back together. Because of these extra red platelets and red blood cells in one place, redness will also be visible in the skin cells surrounding the wound. Once the injury has been closed off from bleeding, and the invading microorganisms have been taken care of, the inflammation response will gradually go down as the skin repairs itself. The swelling and redness will subside, and the skin will lower back to normal body temperature. During this process, the child can go on playing as if nothing had happened. The inflammation won't interrupt his or her daily life while it is present. However, if the inflammation persists and increases where it is no longer needed or appears in an area where there is no damage to repair, it can become a serious problem. This is known as chronic inflammation. This form of inflammation can lead to many health issues, not only depression and anxiety. Examples of these health issues are: Autoimmune diseases such as arthritis, metabolic syndrome, Crohn's disease, and fibromyalgia.

Chronic inflammation happens when the inflammatory response happens frequently, persists long after it is helpful, or even appears unnecessarily. When chronic inflammation develops, the body's immune system can no longer identify the antigens that mark the body's cells as its own. When The white blood cells now view the body's natural cells as invading microorganisms such as harmful bacteria. When this happens, the white blood cells will attack an area of the body as if the cells there were foreign invaders. This problem is known as autoimmune disease. Imagine needing a fist-full of immune system-boosting supplements as a part of every breakfast. Perhaps having a perfectly rehearsed speech about the importance of refraining from contact with you if the other person is or sick, has been sick recently or has recently been in contact with a sick person. Needing physical therapy on your joints and requiring a cane to get around at a young age. This is the daily life of someone with an autoimmune disease. When a person has an autoimmune disease, their body is more susceptible to bacteria and viruses that can cause illness and infections. This is because the immune system is preoccupied with fighting the healthy, body cells and isn't focusing on the real intruders. A person with an autoimmune disease will come down with a cold or flu more often than someone without it, and these common illnesses can be much more dangerous for them. If the immune system isn't taking care of the bacteria or virus that has inflicted the body, they will multiply at a faster rate than they would have otherwise. While this is happening, the white blood cells are also damaging the body which will bring this person down even more. The affected person would have to take special care to avoid others who may be sick and take extra precautions with injuries to avoid sickness and infections at all times. This can create a strain on a person's social life and limit activities that the person can perform. As time goes on and the immune system attacks certain areas of the body, they become increasingly more damaged. Depending on where the unneeded inflammation occurs most often, different problems can arise such as heart disease and cancer. If the immune system continues to attack one place, such as a specific organ, that organ can become seriously damaged. Cancer on the area can form, or the organ may not function properly. Even when it can function, it might be minimally. The best way to prevent these problems is to know how they occur and how they can be slowed or stopped before they get this far. Once an autoimmune disease or arthritis has developed, the damage is generally irreversible. The best action is to take preventative measures and reduce inflammation as much as possible before these health problems begin.

Arthritis, a type of autoimmune disease, happens when the body's immune system triggers the inflammatory response where no injury or foreign organic body is present. The area affected can be anywhere, and, depending on where it occurs, different problems can emerge. In the case of rheumatoid arthritis, the response usually occurs around joints such as knuckles, elbows, or knees. When this happens, the joints can become stiff, swollen, and movement will be painful due to the damage their cells endure from prolonged contact with the now hostile white blood cells. Over time, the damage persists, and more symptoms such as frequent fatigue and fevers can arise. These cells will gather together and build up around the joint. Eventually, they will develop a fibrous layer around the area. Because of this, the joints will erode down much more quickly than normal due to the gathering of inflammatory cells. The pain can become too great to use the joints regularly, eventually crippling them. Physical therapy can be done to help slow the process down and help to maintain mobility, but it only delays the damage. It doesn't remove the cause entirely.

Metabolic syndrome is a collection of risk factors within a single person. Examples of these risk factors are obesity, high blood pressure, high bad cholesterol, and low good cholesterol. If someone has at least three of these factors, they are considered to have metabolic syndrome. Two problems can contribute to, and make metabolic syndrome worse. Insulin resistance and a pro-inflammatory diet. Insulin resistance can be caused by unhealthy eating or high consumption of "diet" labeled foods. How these diet foods create insulin resistance will be broken down and explained in more detail later in this book. Essentially, diet products create an overproduction of insulin. Because metabolic syndrome is a series of mostly diet-related health concerns, the best combatant of it is a change in diet. A shift from trans-fat-rich foods that are packed with sodium and simple sugars to be specific. The best diet option will be explained in more detail as the book continues. The book will also explain how the anti-inflammation can affect hormones such as insulin, and the body's health such as the high blood pressure, and the obesity risk factors that determine if a person has metabolic syndrome. In short, eating whole, healthy foods and limiting or eliminating foods that are high in trans-fat, refined sugars, and salts, and are highly processed is the key to reversing these factors. As most are caused by these unhealthy foods. High blood pressure can happen when the blood is too thick from a concentrated salt and sugar content as well as clogged arteries from trans-fat build-up. Obesity can be countered by a lower intake of calories and consuming these calories in the form of healthy foods as well as a more active lifestyle. Unlike the other diseases, metabolic syndrome can be eliminated by this diet change. However, a failure to do so can result in the development of other diseases.

Crohn's disease is a disease that appears as severe chronic inflammation anywhere in the gastrointestinal tract. Symptoms of Crohn's disease include frequent diarrhea, fever, rectal bleeding from where the intestines meet the anus, stomach ulcers, abdominal cramps, a shortage of energy, fatigue, and a loss of appetite that leads to dramatic weight loss. Where the inflammation is occurring often determines what symptoms appear. For instance, blockages and rectal bleeding are more likely to occur if the inflammation is localized in the intestinal portion of the tract. Some all-around symptoms can show up as well, however. Examples include scar tissue, infections, fistulas which are tubes that can form abnormally within the body between two structures, fissures, which are small tears, and vitamin and mineral deficiencies. Though the location of Crohn's disease is the GI tract, other problems within other areas of the body may occur. The inflammation can spread to the eyes, the skin, and weight can be either dramatically added or reduced without the person actively trying to change it. Though this disease is often caused by genetics and environmental factors, diet serves a very important purpose to a person who has it. Consuming healthy, anti-inflammatory foods can help calm the painful flare-ups that many with this disease suffer. A diet that consists of unhealthy foods can not only cause these painful flare-ups, but it can also make them worse and make them appear more frequently.

Fibromyalgia, another health concern caused by or worsened by chronic inflammation, is a pain disorder that can come with chronic fatigue and mood problems. When a person has fibromyalgia, the nerves within the body send incorrect messages to the brain. The brain processes these messages as pain, which is then felt throughout the body. Those who suffer from fibromyalgia often report the pain as widespread, meaning it is coming from everywhere and on both sides of the body. This pain can feel musculoskeletal. However, the cause isn't the skeleton or the muscles within the body. It feels this way because the pain is simply everywhere and nowhere at the same time as no actual pain is occurring. And though they often sleep for long periods of time, a person with this disorder will feel frequently drained and tired. This is likely because of two factors. Pain on a constant level can be exhausting to deal with, both mentally and physically. It wears on the mind and makes concentration difficult. This can lead to more stress than the initial inflammation even creates, which causes fatigue as well. Also, if the body feels like it is constantly in pain, it will interrupt sleeping patterns as it flares up. If a person can't sleep a constant seven to nine hours a night, they won't feel well rested when they are awake. Fibromyalgia often comes with its own set of symptoms to go along with it. A notable one is irritable bowel syndrome, which will be explained in more detail later in the chapter. Simply, intestinal complications are often linked to both the brain and the person's mood. Both of which are affected by this pain disorder. Multiple occurrences can cause fibromyalgia. Surgeries, chronic inflammation, physical traumas, and psychological stress are all factors that can lead to fibromyalgia. Often, it is a combination of multiple occurrences that lead to the pain disorder, not a single cause. If a person lives with fibromyalgia, chronic inflammation can greatly worsen their symptoms and cause more flare-ups. Because of the extra problems that can arise from chronic inflammation, fibromyalgia included, consuming a diet of anti-inflammatory foods is essential to living with the least amount of pain.

Many factors lead to chronic inflammation. Examples are toxic molds, pollutants, and tobacco products. The most common factor, however, is the diet. When a person's diet consists mostly of unhealthy, pro-inflammatory foods, health complications such as dysbiosis arise. Dysbiosis is caused by a shortage of helpful probiotics and a surplus of harmful bacteria and yeasts in the gastrointestinal, or GI, tract. The bacteria and yeasts necessary to the health of the GI tract also play important roles in the immune system, as well as the brain's functions and even one's personality traits. These bacteria and yeasts can send their own communication signals to the brain the same way neurons electrically send signals such as pain receptors when someone touches a hot plate or whether or not the berry picked straight from the bush tastes like a berry or old beer. These microbes can also help develop important hormones that determine a person's mood such as serotonin. When such an off-balance occurs, a chain reaction begins. Hormonal imbalances, rheumatoid arthritis, cancers, and diseases can appear. Often the symptoms of this disruption are treated, as they are more visible on the outside than the original bacterial imbalance. However, if the root of the problem isn't addressed, the problems will only persist. Foods that contain natural anti-inflammatory properties, such as fish or raw vegetables, can counteract this chronic inflammation, and the decrease in unhealthy foods will allow the GI tract to restore balance to the vital bacteria. The best way to combat chronic inflammation is to begin with the stomach.

Someone who is regularly consuming foods that are high in fiber, phytonutrients, which are the antioxidants found in plant-foods like fruits and vegetables, vitamins, healthy fats, and complex carbohydrates will naturally lower their body's inflammation. Someone else, who chooses to eat processed foods filled with trans-fats, preservatives, and simple sugars, will increase their inflammatory response which will lead to, and increase chronic inflammation. Lacking the filtration effect fiber has on the GI tract and the nutrients provided in vegetables and fruits, as well as natural protein will jump-start the body into a swift, downward spiral. Consuming an unhealthy diet on a regular basis can lead to depression, heart disease, Alzheimer's disease, hormone problems such as PCOS in women, and hypothyroidism, excess fatty tissues that can clog arteries, and dehydration are just a few examples. Because a person's diet is the key factor in producing or removing chronic inflammation developed his anti-inflammation diet. Because the foods it consists of all contain natural anti-inflammatory properties, the diet naturally decreases inflammation in the body and helps maintain healthy hormone, and probiotic levels. With this diet, inflammation as well as the health risks that arise due to it, can be significantly lowered until it is fully focusing on what it should be doing: protecting the body from infections and illnesses.

Why not just take prescribed anti-inflammatory drugs? Well, like any chemically created medication, anti-inflammatory drugs come with their own sets of side effects and complications. People who have taken these medications have an increase in the chances of ulcers in the stomach, shortness of breath if they are allergic, internal bleeding, kidney failure, and liver failure, though it is rare that the liver fails as well. They can also lower the immune system's effectiveness when healing injuries. Instances, an injury such as a bone fracture could take longer to heal than it should if the injured person is taking such medications. It can also heal incorrectly, which an orthodontic surgeon would then need to rebreak and set the bones to heal properly. This especially occurs in those who take anti-inflammatory drugs frequently. The best way to avoid or limit chronic inflammation is by a natural means. And the best way to do that is by consuming anti-inflammatory foods found in the diet.

Chapter 2:
The History and Science
of the Anti-Inflammation Diet

All of the diseases and health complications mentioned in chapter one are different branches that connect to the same root. Inflammation. As also discussed in chapter one, chemically produced medications taken to decrease inflammation in the body can harm it in their own ways. When it comes to chronic inflammation, a change in lifestyle can go a long way to alleviate or sometimes even eliminate negative symptoms of these health concerns. Nutrition and fitness play a key role in how inflammation affects the mind and body. Explained in this chapter is how and why the anti-inflammation diet was developed, what it consists of, and how best to create foods that will ultimately improve all aspects of life. If the body isn't getting the nutrients and exercise it needs to function optimally, it won't run without some problems. This diet is easy to follow, isn't restrictive on calorie-intake or food categories beyond health, and is inclusive of all tastes and cultures.

As mentioned before, the anti-inflammation, or the anti-inflammatory diet, was developed by Dr. Andrew Weil. Weil was a student at Harvard University and studied integrative medicine. Integrative medicine, unlike more common practices, is a medicinal technique that works to improve the whole person, both physically and mentally, and not just the medical problem visible at that time. Integrative medicine focuses on improving the health and function of the physical body, as well as the mind and psychological state. Weil aimed to prevent chronic inflammation-induced health problems such as heart disease, rheumatoid arthritis, and Alzheimer's disease using a method that would seek the original problem that caused the chronic inflammation in the first place. Without the root problem, the rest of the complications will ease. And because the main factor that contributes to chronic inflammation is unhealthy eating habits, his solution was to develop the anti-inflammation diet. His diet focuses on consuming the anti-inflammatory properties in some foods and avoiding the chemicals that could lead to more inflammation in others. However, the aim of the diet doesn't only counter inflammation. Weil developed a balanced diet that adds nutrition, health and doesn't require a severely low-calorie intake. When a person's diet consists mostly of fast food, their bodies will obtain mostly preservatives, unhealthy amounts of sodium, simple carbohydrates, and unhealthy fats. The meat is generally highly processed, and the wheat products are typically simple white carbohydrates. When eaten on a regular basis, the body lacks nutrition that it needs to run smoothly. The trans-fat builds up in the blood vessels, and the high sodium content creates problems for the heart and kidneys. The simple sugars and carbs will quickly spike and then dramatically drop the blood sugar levels. The preservatives and chemicals put into the food can create problems in the GI tract by upsetting the balance of good and bad bacteria that reside there and create problems for the liver and kidneys that filter it out. The excess sugars, salts, and fats provide inflammatory properties.

Processed food is food that has been prepared with preservatives and made into a simple, easy-to-prepare form. Though convenient, processed food is packed full of unhealthy, and often unnatural ingredients. Preservatives are added to prolong the shelf-life, or how long the food can remain in the store before it isn't legally sellable. These preservatives are chemicals that are difficult for the liver to break down and filter out of the body. No two are alike. However, each is harmful in a different way. Generally, they can cause several health complications. Examples of these complications are trouble breathing, different kinds of cancer, heart damage and a change in behavior such as hyperactivity, especially in young children. Often these foods are filled with sodium chloride, which is the common table salt. Sodium chloride is not a natural salt. It is heavily processed to remove minerals that can be beneficial to the body, such as the minerals found in sea salt or Himalayan pink salt. Chemicals are added to sodium chloride to prevent clumping, which is visually appealing and makes using it easier. However, these chemicals are just as harmful as preservatives. Another common ingredient in these foods is simple, bleached sugar. All fruits and carbohydrates have natural sugars, both of which are necessary to a balanced diet. Processed sugars, however, are full of these same harmful chemicals and tend to cause grogginess and fatigue after consumption. They also cause a dramatic, but short-lived, rise in the blood sugar, then an equally dramatic drop that can last hours. The problem with these processed foods is that nearly everything found in a store has them. Unless food is bought in raw or comes from a reliable source, it likely contains these harmful preservatives. The best way to safely avoid them is to buy whole ingredients to prepare a meal and not convenient, packaged goods.

When such unhealthy food is consumed, the body and mind are both affected. Excessive sodium found in many unhealthy foods dramatically shifts the water content in the body. Because water flows toward solids, such as salt, through porous membranes, such as the stomach or intestines, it will follow the sodium that travels through the body. The body will become dehydrated. The kidneys function to remove waste products by filtering it out with water out of the body. If the body is dehydrated, the kidneys will have to quickly sort out how much water to hold onto and how much can be filtered through to remove wastes. Without enough proper hydration, these wastes cannot be removed, and if they build up too much, they can harm the body. Often, instead of drinking water or tea to balance out this problem, soft drinks follow the high salt intake. These drinks are composed of mostly high fructose corn syrup, which is a very unhealthy form of thick sugar that is illegal to put into food or drinks in most other countries. The intake increases these solids as the sugars are introduced into the body which will dehydrate the body further. These unhealthy chemicals are now both the kidneys' problem and the liver as well. The body must work extra hard to filter these out and try to hold onto as much water as possible. The body is composed of 70% water, so such dehydration can cause problems such as kidney stones, migraines, and even some shrinking in the brain. The sugars present in these kinds of foods will drop the blood sugar levels at the same time. Put together, the body will feel extremely heavy and fatigued, dehydrated, the stomach will feel heavy with all of the trans-fats, and headaches will occur all at once. This is only the immediate consequence of eating these foods. The long-term effects are an even greater concern.

If such a diet persists, the body will wear down at a much faster rate than it should. Some parts will do so faster than others. The most common problem that comes up from high sodium and trans-fats is heart disease. The fatty tissues that build up in arteries can create a much higher blood pressure as the heart must push harder and more frequently to keep the blood going through these smaller tunnels. The excess salt content in the blood and the extra water that cannot be lost creates thicker blood. Combined with the now thinner blood vessels, this creates a very serious strain on the heart that will persist until the food intake is changed, and the fat build-up removed. The heart is both a muscle and an organ. As a vital organ, it cannot rest or the whole cardiovascular system will shut down. This would lead to death within minutes, as blood carries oxygen from the lungs to every cell in the body. Without oxygen, the cells will die. As a muscle, frequent and difficult work can wear out the heart and eventually cause heart attacks or even failure. If enough excess fat builds up around the lungs and on the chest, it can cause sleep apnea and trouble breathing as the fatty tissues collected create a smaller space for the lungs to expand. In addition to this small space, the tissues also add much more weight that the lungs have to work against when pulling in air. The stomach can develop ulcers from the high fat and salt content, and the esophagus may develop cancerous cells. Excess weight build-up will put pressure on joints; specifically knees and ankles. These are only a few examples, as there are many ways such a diet inhibits the body.

Weil's diet, ranked fourteenth in best overall diets, takes all these factors into careful consideration. It doesn't only replace naturally inflaming foods with anti-inflammatory ones, it also provides only healthy, nutritious food that the body needs to work properly. When fast food or unhealthy food is replaced with natural, raw foods to be prepared for a meal, the body responds accordingly. Healthy fats replace the trans-fats that can severely damage the body. Sodium is significantly lowered, and the healthier food won't bog down the body and mind. The transition could potentially help those with excess weight lose it, especially when coupled with an active lifestyle. Such a lifestyle is also recommended by Weil, as it produces more endorphins. Endorphins can be explained as "happiness" chemicals in the brain. A boost of endorphins can help fight depression.

The anti-inflammation diet is based on a 2,000-3,000-calorie intake. Of course, this can change based on factors such as age, size, gender, and activity level. The macronutrients, which are protein, fatty acids, and carbohydrates, are what make up the majority of the calorie number. Around 20-30% of these calories should come from protein, 40-50% from complex carbohydrates and 30% from healthy, unsaturated, omega-3 fatty acids. A variety of fruits and vegetables rich in anti-inflammatory properties should also be consumed throughout the day. No less than five cups per day of vegetables, and about three to four cups per day of fruit. A break-down of what foods these qualities consist of is provided below.

When it comes to protein, one size does not fit all. In this diet, choosing the correct foods to satisfy the protein factor is important.

Red meats, such as ground beef and steak are full of animal fats and can contribute to the increase of inflammation. Such fat can be seen dripping from a pizza or pooling in a skillet as the burger is being cooked. Black beans and oily fish are excellent choices that fulfill the protein need. Black beans coupled with brown rice creates the perfect protein to replace meat with. Beans and rice are both incomplete proteins. However, what one is lacking, the other contains. The combination also creates a delicious dinner when seasoned with chili pepper and complemented with a salad or stir-fry. Oily fish contains omega-3 fatty acids, which are crucial to any healthy diet. Fish is a very lean meat packed with protein and vitamin D. A vitamin D deficiency can cause a low mood and even depression. The oils within the fish contribute to the 30% of healthy fats needed in the day. Greek yogurts also contain protein and often are sweetened with fruits. Yogurt also contains helpful probiotics to help provide a boost to the healthy bacteria in the stomach, which is useful, especially when taking antibiotics. Although, it is important to pay attention to the ingredients listed in any packaged product. Any word that rhymes with "gross" is a type of sugar, such as the word "fructose" in high fructose corn syrup. Also, the order of which these ingredients are listed is important. The first word is the ingredient that is most present in the product, and the final ingredient is the least. For example, if glucose is the first word listed in the ingredients, the contents contain mostly sugar. Though a natural sugar is present in all fruits, it would not be listed first without added, unnatural sugars. Avoiding foods like these is important to maintain the anti-inflammation diet.

Perhaps one of the more confusing aspects of Weil's diet is the high amount of fats required. About 30% of the caloric intake should be from fats, and yet fatty foods should be avoided at all costs. The truth is, not all fats are unhealthy like the oil dripping off French fries. There are different kinds of fats, and it is important to understand which are healthy to consume, and which should not even be touched. Animal fats, which provides the moisture in the hamburger patty at a barbeque, is unhealthy fat. Examples of these unhealthy fats are: dark poultry meats which are thighs and legs, fatty pork, beef, and lard. Another unhealthy fat is corn-based vegetable oil. Not to be confused with olive oil, which is an omega-3 rich, healthy fat. Trans-fats can clog arteries and cause heart disease and obesity if consumed regularly. They can also contribute to chronic inflammation, the unhealthy bacteria balance, and the drained feeling after eating. Healthy fats, which contain omega-3 fatty acids, can be found in nuts, avocados, fish oil, and coconut oil. Every cell in the body is composed lipids, which are fatty acids. Without healthy fat, cells cannot regenerate, and the body would be unable to function properly. However, excess fat creates extra cells of fat to be stored for later. During the time of hunting and gathering, these extra cells would provide energy during a long period without food. Now, however, as food is easy to locate, this survival feature can be a problem. When too many of these cells have accumulated, the result is obesity, which leads to several health complications such as type two diabetes, sleep apnea, heart disease and cancer. Healthy fats, when eaten at the correct rates, provide the needed fats for cells, but not in such excess that fat cells form.

When it comes to carbohydrates, the more complex, the better. Simple carbs, such as white rice, and white or simple wheat bread, contain little to no fiber and become simple sugars in the body that harm more than they help. These simple sugars promote inflammation and cause blood sugar to spike and drop dramatically. During the spike, the body will feel over-energized, and the result could lead to anxiety. The drop, however, which occurs very quickly after the spike, is the opposite. The body becomes sluggish and the mind fatigued. Everything feels like too much effort and the bed is inviting. Complex carbs such as quinoa, brown rice, and multigrain bread break down into complex sugars that the body needs. Unlike the simpler sugars, they regulate blood sugar at a constant, normal level to maintain energy throughout the day, and keep the body going. Consuming whole grains is important for the GI tract, as they are packed with fiber that can act as a filtration system in the digestive organs. Fiber also helps flush out waste where unhealthy foods pack it together and keep it immobile. This can cause great discomfort in the bowels. The fiber paired with the anti-inflammatory properties can reduce the unhelpful microorganisms in the stomach and provide more room for the beneficial bacteria to take over.

Vegetables and some fruits can also be high in fiber. They contain vitamins, minerals, and phytonutrients that act as antioxidants, which removes oxidizing agents in the body. Variety is important when it comes to vegetables, as each contains different benefits to the body. Beneficial vegetables include green, leafy vegetables such as romaine lettuce, spinach, and kale, cruciferous vegetables such as cabbage and broccoli, and alliums like leeks and green onions are all different kinds of anti-inflammation vegetables. Not only do they naturally decrease inflammation, but each vegetables has their own health benefit to add. Carrots provide vitamin A which is good for the eyes. Celery is a high-fiber vegetable that is full of water to flush out waste and hydrate. Cauliflower is full of vitamins C, and K. Vitamin C boosts the immune system, while vitamin K helps the blood clot arteries while providing a boost in the healing response. Fruits provide vitamins that are important for body functions. Examples of beneficial fruits are berries like strawberries and raspberries, apples, pineapple, and oranges. Blueberries can benefit the brain function, and memory and oranges are high in essential vitamin C.

Spices are not only helpful for adding flavor to foods, but some even contain their own anti-inflammation benefits. Turmeric, garlic, and chili powder can be added to different dishes to provide both health benefits and flavor. Drinks such as green tea and red wine provide antioxidants and pair well with lunches and dinners. Dark chocolate is a healthy, occasional treat that can be incorporated into Weil's diet. It is also healthy for the heart when consumed in moderation.

Chapter 2: The History and Science of the Anti-Inflammation Diet

General foods that can be found in Weil's anti-inflammation diet include, but are not limited to:

Vegetables:

- Kale
- Spinach
- Romaine lettuce
- Iceberg lettuce
- Tomatoes
- Celery
- Zucchini
- Cauliflower
- Peppers
- Onions
- Green onions
- Leeks
- Snap peas
- Green beans
- Brussel sprouts
- Asparagus
- Squash

Fruits:

- Strawberries
- Passionfruit
- Starfruit

- Raspberries
- Blueberries
- Blackberries
- Huckleberries
- Pineapple
- Apples
- Pears
- Oranges
- Grapes
- Kiwi
- Bananas
- Mango
- Papaya
- Starfruit
- Pomegranate
- Cherries
- Lemons
- Limes
- Honeydew melons
- Cantaloupe

Carbohydrates:

- Brown rice
- Quinoa
- Steel-cut oats
- Multigrain bread

- Oat Flour
- Nuts

Protein:

- Greek yogurt
- Salmon
- Trout
- Chicken breast
- Turkey breast
- Black beans with brown rice
- Egg whites

Fats:

- Olive oil
- Coconut oil
- Avocados
- Peanuts
- Almonds
- Cashews
- Pistachios

Spices:

- Turmeric
- Chili powder
- Black pepper

- Garlic
- Ginger

Supplements:

- Apple cider vinegar
- B-complex vitamins
- Branched-chain amino acids (BCAAs)
- L-Carnitine
- Multivitamins
- Green coffee bean
- Chromium

Other:

- Dark chocolate
- Red wine
- Green tea
- Black tea

Listed within Weil's food pyramid are daily supplements which are usually found in pill form. What supplements a person should take varies based on their own body's needs and outside factors such as the weather. If it is the middle of spring, and the rainclouds have been covering the sun for weeks, a supplement of vitamin D3 might be in order until the rain subsides. Taking BCAAs at night after a particularly strenuous workout can help to build the torn muscle tissues back up more quickly, which will reduce soreness and for how long the muscle is sore. Apple cider vinegar tablets are beneficial to lose weight, maintain blood sugar levels and has many overall health benefits. It's a great supplement for a woman with PCOS who is trying to shed extra pounds. A supplement that everyone should take is a multivitamin. What kind depends on gender and personal circumstance, so it is best to speak to a doctor or nutrition expert on what vitamin combination is best for you. It is also important to know how different supplements can affect the body and brain, as taking some for long periods of time and suddenly stopping, can create a depression dip. Some energy supplements, such as B12 or B6, are important to boosting the immune system, however taking too much too often can wear down the heart just as caffeine can. Knowing your body and how the supplements you are taking work is important. Though supplementing can benefit, doing so incorrectly can cause more harm than good.

Balanced meals are important to maintain the guidelines of the anti-inflammation diet. Below is an example of a day's worth of meals that follow the anti-inflammation diet:

> ➢ Steel cut oats seasoned with cinnamon and honey, with a Greek yogurt side for breakfast.

> ➢ A handful of assorted, unsalted nuts such as peanuts, almonds, and cashews as a snack.

> ➢ A lunch of grilled salmon, with a tossed salad of romaine lettuce, sliced tomatoes, grated carrots, dried cranberries, and a Greek yogurt dressing. Best enjoyed with green tea sweetened with honey.

> ➢ A snack of multigrain toast topped with two slices of avocado.

> ➢ Stir-fried zucchini seasoned with ginger, grilled chicken breast seasoned with garlic and a side of brown rice seasoned with turmeric. Enjoy dinner with a glass of wine.

> ➢ A small piece of dark chocolate after dinner.

It is also important to change up what meals are being prepared. Different ingredients can add different nutrients, vitamins, and benefits to the body. Even simply replacing the zucchini with green peppers, onions, and spinach or eating egg whites on toast with a side of sliced apples for breakfast instead of the steel-cut oats. Consuming the same meals each day will limit the body and can become tedious and unsatisfying over time. If someone isn't feeling satisfaction from taste, or excitement from trying something new, the temptation to stray from the diet all together can be difficult to resist. To avoid sneaking unhealthy foods and feeling guilty for it later, try recipes found on health-food sites or cookbooks, or even experiment to see what textures and flavors create the best dishes. Removing unhealthy food doesn't have to feel like a punishment. It's a chance to be adventurous in the kitchen and create a more fulfilling life while you're at it!

These days, many people are busy with work, errands, family, or other engagements that can take up most their time. It's difficult to juggle work, family, friends, personal time and health all in one. This problem is why convenient and unhealthy foods can become such a problem as quickly as they have. It's much easier to grab something at a drive through on the way to work than to prepare a meal. Though, an understandable situation, there are always other options available. One only has to find them. One way to overcome such a busy life is by cooking ahead of time, or making extra food when there is time to cook, and portioning it out. Portioning food is when the calorie need is calculated to figure out how much food should be consumed at a time and storing that amount in a container. Setting aside one for each day of the week creates a quick, portable meal that can easily be heated up when needed. If the food is ready to go and prepared ahead of time, it can be picked up on the way out the door. It's even faster than a drive-thru, therefore, more convenient too! A sample menu for foods that can be prepared are:

> A baked turkey sliced into meat for sandwiches.

> Stuffed peppers made with anti-inflammatory vegetables and spices, spices, brown rice, and shredded chicken breast.

> Salads that have been put together ahead of times. Prolonged contact with dressing can make the lettuce soggy, so store it separately until the day of.

> Baby carrots, sliced celery, cauliflower florets, and chopped broccoli with a home-maid, Greek yogurt vegetable dip.

> Brown rice, steamed vegetables, and grilled fish.

> Whole grain pasta with a cauliflower sauce base.

> A fruit salad with Greek yogurt and nuts.

> Casseroles made with whole ingredients.

Knowing the calorie count in each ingredient in a meal is important to determine how much to eat in a sitting. If bought as separate ingredients, it is possible to calculate each by how many calories are in the ingredient. There are sites specifically designed to calculate calories, so inputting how much of each ingredient was used is all you need to do to know. Once the count is calculated, you can determine how much food should be made to satisfy the calorie amount. If the food product is bought in a package by a trusted source, calorie information can be found on the nutrition label at the top, left-hand corner. However, it is important to understand how those labels are meant to be read. The calorie amount listed is based on the serving size, which isn't always the exact amount within the package, or the amount you'll expect. For instance, one slice of bread is considered a single serving size, not two. So if two slices were consumed in a sandwich, the calorie count found on the label is only half of the actual amount of the meal. It's always a good idea to double-check, or use a search engine if you're unsure, as the calorie amount can determine the best fitness actions to take, and how much to eat at a given time.

Any diet transition can be difficult when unhealthy foods are full of addictive properties such as preservatives, salts, and simple sugars. When a strong craving hits, it is possible to make a healthier version of the desired food. It can sometimes take a little creativity, but it is usually possible after some experimentation. For example, sliced eggplant, when baked can create a crust-like texture. Topped with a home-made tomato sauce and lean turkey sausage, it can become a small, healthy pizza. Burritos can be made with shredded chicken breast, homemade salsa, cumin, and a whole grain wrap. Plain, Greek yogurt can supplement for sour cream to top them off. Steamed cauliflower, when blended with a splash of milk can become a creamy sauce for pasta. Add some Greek yogurt, garlic, and onion powder to top over brown rice noodles to create an alfredo dinner. Frozen bananas can be blended and refrozen to form a base for a healthy ice cream replacement. If a strong pasta craving hits, but there is no more room for carbohydrates for the day, replacing the noodles with zucchini noodles, or zoodles can satisfy it. Experimenting in the kitchen can make the anti-inflammation diet fun and add variety.

Provided are a few examples:

➢ Ground turkey sausage instead of pork sausage

➢ Arrowroot instead of cornstarch

➢ Sunflower butter instead of dairy butter

➢ Oat flour instead of bleached flour

➢ Honey instead of sugar

> ➢ Blended cauliflower instead of mashed potatoes

> ➢ Zucchini noodles instead of flour

> ➢ Pure maple instead of brown sugar

Many ingredients can supplement unhealthy ones that aren't listed, because it takes creativity, at times, to discover what works well and what doesn't. Finding what healthy foods can behave like unhealthy foods can be tricky at times, but a part of the fun is experimentation and learning as you go. That veggie burger may not have stayed together very well without egg yolk, but it might work the next time with a different ingredient. Those pancakes that were made from Greek yogurt, oat flour, and egg whites may have come out stiff and leathery, so perhaps adding a little milk and water would make it better next time. There are also many different recipes for food swapping in cookbooks or found online. There's a way to make a favorite, unhealthy dish out of only healthy ingredients out there. One simply needs to find them and put them to use.

Chapter 3:
Health Benefits and Connections to Depression, Stress, and Anxiety

Mental health concerns such as depression and anxiety can make life difficult and exhausting. This chapter will explain the connections between chronic inflammation and stress, as well as how they two can work together to become even worse. It will discuss what aspects of chronic inflammation can contribute to depression and anxiety, as well as hormonal complications such as PCOS in women and diabetes. Also within this chapter is the importance of a healthy diet when someone suffers mental illnesses, and how the anti-inflammation diet can counter the rise of cortisol with inflammation, raise the overall mood and how to combat the vicious cycle of stress eating with examples of healthy ways to combat stress. The benefits of adding fitness to your lifestyle and your change of diet provide an extra boost that can restore energy throughout the day, create endorphins in the brain and generate an overall better lifestyle for the body and mind will be described and explained within this chapter.

As mentioned before, the healthy bacteria in the GI tract are both connected to the immune system as well as many hormone systems in the body. One hormone, serotonin, is found in blood platelets as well as the GI tract. When the tract is inflamed, serotonin levels in the body will drop. Many antidepressants work to bring serotonin levels back up to normal. However, if the GI tract remains inflamed, the root cause has not been addressed, and the problem will continue. When it comes to stress and its connection to mation, a cycle can begin. Chronic stress, which can come from PTSD, residing in a stressful living situation, constant overexertion, or working a stressful and unfulfilling job, can trigger inflammation in the GI tract, and inflammation in the GI tract can release cortisol. Cortisol is the stress hormone, which is released when a stressful situation occurs. It is helpful in situations of an attack, as the response is meant to provide an extra burst of energy to flee or fight. However, the cortisol response is unhealthy at a constant rate. Unfortunately, it cannot judge between a nervous reaction and a literally life-threatening circumstance. For instance, if someone is at an important job interview, but they spill coffee on their white shirt just before the hiring manager meets with them, cortisol levels will spike just as they would if someone were to threaten that person for their money. Because of this direct connection between the GI tract and cortisol, stress, and chronic inflammation work hand-in-hand as each brings the other up. The cortisol will trigger an inflammatory response, which will then trigger more cortisol. This cycle can go on and increasingly get worse if it continues unchecked. Luckily, this same connection works by bringing both down. When consuming a diet of anti-inflammation foods, the inflammation levels will go down, and these hormones can return to regular levels.

Research has found that consuming foods high in trans-fat and sodium can increase depression at a shocking rate of 58%! In multiple studies volunteers without prior depression changed their diet from anti-inflammatory to pro-inflammatory foods that were high in fats, simple sugars, and sodium. After the three-year-long study was over, most of the volunteers reported feeling much more prone to depression and anxiety. People with preexisting depression and anxiety who had switched from unhealthy foods to omega-3 oils, fresh meat, instead of processed meats, and vegetables were less likely to experience depression or anxiety. Each study suggested that the unhealthy, fatty foods triggered an inflammatory response in the body that started the chain reaction of health complications.

Chapter 3: Health Benefits and Connections to Depression, Stress, and Anxiety

The inflammation isn't the only problem these foods cause, however. The refined and false sugars commonly found in "diet" foods and highly processed foods can cause insulin resistance in the body, which has been linked to major depression, and Polycystic Ovarian Syndrome (PCOS) in women, diabetes and metabolic syndrome. Low energy, inflammation, and insulin resistance can all combine to major depression and anxiety that wouldn't have occurred before.

If a prepackaged product is labeled as "diet," it isn't actually a part of any healthy diet. The word diet, in this context, actually means that the sugar ingredient was switched out for a chemical supplement. This chemical is actually even more harmful to the body in different ways than even the simple sugars. Insulin will be produced as this false sugar enters the body. Because insulin can only break down real sugars, this diet sugar cannot be processed. The insulin has nothing to do and remains in the body, making it groggy and tired. When real sugars are consumed, such as that found in fruit, even more, insulin is produced to break that down, leaving the original wave with no job to do except exist. Eventually, this will create an insulin resistance in the body. Issues such as the inability to remain awake and falling asleep at inappropriate times will arise, and PCOS can develop.

Imagine a woman coming home from a ten-hour long shift cooking at a restaurant. It's been a busy day, and the line of customers was out the door the whole shift. When she gets home, her children are yelling and creating chaos out of the house. Once she has wrestled her children into bed, the woman might sneak into the dark kitchen and look for a pint of ice cream she had saved just for nights like these. She breaks up her favorite candy bar and sprinkles it over the generous bowl of ice cream and dishes in. This situation is known as stress-eating. The problem with stress eating is that commercially baked goods and unhealthy foods can cause even more stress on top of the other health problems they are known to cause. Because of the spike and drop from simple sugars and carbohydrates, they will become anxious for a short time and then fatigued after their binge. The lack of motivation will lead to more stress as responsibilities are ignored, which can lead to even more stress eating. As this cycle continues, the junk food being eaten adds up to several health problems in the heart, liver, kidneys, stomach, and brain. The cycle adds up and takes its own toll on the body and mind. The stress alone can lead to anxiety and depression and weakens the immune system, which will already have its own complications due to the inflammation occurring from the unhealthy foods. As mentioned previously, chronic stress can contribute to chronic inflammation that will lead to a rise in cortisol which is the stress hormone. As the eating habit continues, so too does the stress it is meant to be alleviating.

Such stress can lead to anxiety, but it isn't the only factor causing the panic attacks that keep people inside. That same spike and drop that can lead to depression can also be a factor for anxiety. The initial spike in blood sugar provides a rush of energy much like caffeine or energy drinks. This energy burst can create an anxious, revved-up feeling that will develop into or increase existing anxiety. Coupled with stress-eating habits, this anxious feeling can make it difficult to concentrate or get involved in social situations. Isolation from friends or family can contribute to more depression, and the inability to concentrate can create even more stress. The inflammation resulting from these foods, and the hormone imbalances that occur from the inflammation will make their own contributions to these mental health concerns. Hormones are responsible for many responses in the body. A hormone called insulin breaks down consumed sugars and processes them to be used in the body. The pituitary gland in the brain secretes growth hormones so that a child will grow into an adult. Hormones are responsible for emotions as well as a person's responses to them. When the eaten junk food inflames the body, and these hormones are thrown off balance, the body cannot cope as well with stress.

Serotonin can decrease, and hormonal complications may appear. When someone develops a hormone imbalance, emotions can become out of control the way women are known to feel more emotional when pregnant. They can also lead to more physical complications, which are often stressful to cope with.

There are a few ways to combat the stress-eating habit. Finding a new coping mechanism for stress, such as journaling or going for a walk, are healthy habits that will also benefit in some other way. Eating green, leafy vegetables instead of junk food may satisfy the physical motion of the stress-eating habit without compromising the body's health. Because green vegetables contain very few calories, they can be eaten in large quantities without any negative consequences. And since lettuce or spinach has little to no flavor, eating may become boring over time, and the desire will be decreased. Even if it doesn't, sitting down on the couch and eating a bowl of shredded lettuce while watching a comedy is much healthier than if the bowl contained assorted candies. In addition to changing up the foods that are being eaten to cope with stress, trying out other mechanisms can help lower stress levels. Examples of other activities are taking a hot bath with bubbles or relaxing salts, aromatherapy oils in a the bath or a diffuser, soothing music, going for a walk around the neighborhood, taking a class such as a painting or pottery class after work, any kinds of exercise, talking with someone, or a hot cup of herbal tea.

A recent study found a significant connection between the gut microbes and the mood as well as psychological functions. The study found that, if a change were made to the microbes in the gut, a change in one's mental state would occur as a result. The researches named the causes of these changes psychobiotics. Psychobiotics can be both beneficial and detrimental to the mind and body. Positive psychobiotics, such as the anti-inflammation diet, exercise, and the probiotics found in Greek yogurt, can elevate the mood, and decrease the risk for diseases. Psychobiotics such as antibiotics and fast food decrease the amount of helpful gut microbes and can lead to more health problems and depression. The study is new, so there isn't an over-the-counter pill that can balance out the healthy and unhealthy microbes in the GI tract. However, following the anti-inflammation diet, eating plenty of Greek yogurt while on antibiotics, and exercise are all natural, positive psychobiotics that can be incorporated into daily life.

An unfortunate truth is that taking antibiotics when needed is not avoidable. If a serious infection or illness occurs that won't heal alone, it could spread to other parts of the body and become a serious health risk. When such an infection occurs, a doctor may prescribe an antibiotic to clear it away and potentially prevent serious illness or death, depending on the severity of the infection or bacterial illness at that time. Antibiotics are designed to attack all bacteria in the body to remove harmful, invading microbes. Unfortunately, the healthy gut microbes often get caught up in the mix and are eliminated as well. Regardless, neglecting to take prescribed antibiotics is not the answer, as they are potentially life-saving and help prevent spreading the infection to other people. There are different options of probiotics that can be ingested while on antibiotics to help replace what the medication has eliminated. Yogurt is the most common example. Because it is naturally full of probiotics, doctors will often recommend an increased intake of yogurt, preferably Greek yogurt, while someone is taking antibiotics. Sauerkraut and dark chocolate are less well-known examples of probiotic foods that can restore the healthy microbes. Though certainly helpful and necessary, there is more that can be done in addition to eating probiotic-rich foods to keep the gut healthy when taking antibiotics. Maintaining the anti-inflammation diet and exercise will not only help to replace the microbes, but it will also maintain a healthy immune system that can attack invading bacteria before it becomes a serious infection more successfully.

Other than diet, exercise is one of the most important psychobiotics to a daily routine. Not only does it work with the diet to reduce inflammation and improve overall health, but it also decreases sarcopenia. Sarcopenia is the naturally-occurring muscle deterioration that happens with age. However, it isn't natural to occur at an accelerated rate in a young person. Chronic inflammation can speed up the sarcopenia process in the body, which leads to weakened muscles and fatigue. A minimum of thirty minutes of exercise per day can slow down or even stop the process of sarcopenia with the combined use of the anti-inflammation diet. It can also increase endorphins in the brain, balance out gut microbes, keep the heart and lungs healthy, and provide energy for the day. All these factors add up to an elevated mood and a decrease in depression. Switching up cardio and body weight exercises can build muscle tone, increase stamina, and boost confidence in addition to the health benefits it can bring. Not all exercise has to be at the gym. If an at-home workout is more comfortable, there are plenty to be found online to stream, and there is a surplus of video fitness programs that can be purchased. Dancing, martial arts, yoga, circuits, and Pilates are all examples of different types of workouts that can take the place of the typical gym's treadmill and bench press workout. Going for a jog around town or going on a hike in the woods are great cardio options. When on a treadmill, the surface is level, and the track is straight ahead. When jogging on a track, around a neighborhood, or around a park involved running on less even ground, will help to improves balance. Being able to meander and turn will improve coordination. Mixing up a workout routine can keep it exciting and work different muscle groups to maintain a strong body overall. For example, you could go with a dance routine on Monday, some bodyweight exercises the next day, a jog on Wednesday, upper body heavy lifting on Thursday, yoga on Friday, lower body heavy lifting on Saturday, and martial arts on Sunday. The possibilities are endless, and the increase in activity can provide a personal challenge every day. You could time yourself on a jog, or aim for one more push-up before muscle failure. Setting goals will also help you stay with it and work to be better each day.

Chapter 4:
The Connection Between Intestinal and Mental Health

Inflammation and gut bacteria are often linked when it comes to medical complications. Because gut microbes play such a vital role in how a body and mind function, it is important to understand them, what outside factors can affect a change in their population within the gut, how an imbalance of these microbes can affect mental health, and what studies are being done to learn more about them. Explained within the chapter is how gut microbes communicate with the brain and body, and why different types are vital to different brain functions such as social interaction. Also explained will be the connection between autism and inflammation, as well as autism and gut microbes. This example of how chronic inflammation, gut health, and mental health are all intertwined in one mess of health, and how much science really understands about this connection in recent studies.

The common phrases "Gut feeling" and "Butterflies in the stomach" are more accurate than many might think. The GI tract is connected to, and sensitive to the emotions felt within the body. There is a very tangible connection between the brain and the GI tract. For example, if someone who had accidentally eaten rotten yogurt at one time in their life thinks about or sees some yogurt later on, they will feel nauseous in the stomach and a loss of appetite. If a person is hungry, the brain will let the stomach know to feel hungry as a way of making someone seek out nutrients. And if that hungry person thinks about a savory chicken breast, the stomach will know and ce more digestive enzymes in preparation for the food. Because of this connection, the brain and GI tract can affect each other. Much like the inflammation response and its connection with cortisol levels, mental health and the gut can bring each other down and up. If one is healthy, often, so is the other.

There are multiple ways microbes can communicate with the brain. Two examples are the enteric nervous system and the vagus nerve. The enteric nervous system, which is an intricate subdivision of the nervous system, controls parts of the endocrine system, as well as the GI tract. The endocrine system is responsible for hormone control and production within the body. Hormones such as serotonin and cortisol can help deliver messages from the microbes to the brain. Other microbes might evolve to connect with the brain via the vagus nerve, which is a nerve connection between the gut and the brain. Because of this intricate connection, any small offset in the balance can create a chain reaction within the whole body and mind. Hormones are often the cause or indication of a mental and physical complications. Low serotonin can cause depression, a surplus of the growth hormone can force a person to grow too large for their heart to pump blood to their whole body effectively, and low estrogen in women can cause infertility, irregular cycles and change their voice. If there is a problem within the gut, and the microbes that communicate to the brain using the enteric system are missing or low, these problems may present themselves. A study was done with mice to see just how important these microbes are to mental health.

In a lab study, mice were bred in an anti-bacterial environment. As they grew older, they displayed signs of mental and physical health problems. The other mice, which were bred in a more natural, germy environment, did display these patterns of behavior. Lacking the natural microbes that reside in the GI tract seemed to cause social confusion in the germ-free mice. After interacting with other rates, they seemed to forget them. Their behavior matched that of a mouse greeting someone new each time they met with another mouse they had previously seen. Gut microbes naturally need to spread to other living bodies to multiply and grow as a species of living organism. So, as a survival mechanism, they have evolved to communicate with the social part of the brain and create the desire to interact with and remember others of the same species. Because of the connection between the brain and these microbes, the mice that were missing these microbes were antisocial and did not recognize a familiar face no matter how many times they were introduced. Also, these same mice also seemed to behave in a way similar to humans who suffer from depression, anxiety, autism, and chronic stress. Once the strains of the missing microbes were introduced into the GI tract of these mice, their symptoms faded or, in some cases, went away altogether. These findings led scientists to believe that adding certain probiotics to the treatment of a depressed patient could be the key to help them overcome their depression. Though probiotics alone aren't enough. Other psychobiotics such as the anti-inflammation diet and physical activity together provide the gut with the essential microbes responsible for countering depression and anxiety.

Scientists also noted another interesting connection between the GI tract and the brain. When extracting the fecal bacteria a curious, social mouse curious and introducing it into the stomach of a naturally timid mouse, he may become more curious and social. When microbes from an anxious mouse were introduced in a calm mouse's GI tract, signs of anxiety would begin to show as he would become restless. This discovery explains the role that bacteria and yeasts in the GI tract play on a personality. Their connection to the brain drives personality traits and emotions that the brain is known to be responsible for. A person born with one trait and another person born with a different trait will also be born with different probiotics in their guts. This study suggests that introducing certain microbes into someone's gut could potentially alter the person's whole personality. If isolated, traits such as mood disorders, depression, bad temper, and anxiety could eventually be changed or removed. The study is new, and the technology to do so doesn't exist yet, but the discovery is a step in the right direction.

Another notable connection between the GI tract and the brain is the effect intestinal illnesses will have on a person's mental state. People known to have intestinal illnesses tend to also have psychological symptoms that they may not be able to explain. A person who has no prior history of mental health complications that might come down with irritable bowel syndrome might experience an increase of depression at the time of being sick. The same person may later experience a chest cold without the same effect. This would suggest the mental symptom wasn't caused by general illness. This also explains why a person may experience the need for a restroom when feeling nervous or anxious. The mood of nervousness will trigger irritation in the stomach and intestines. This will cause upset stomach and irritable bowels at the time the emotion occurs. Following a theory that a mother's body temperature and whether a constant fever could cause a child to be born autistic, a man named Dr. Paul Patterson, studied a pregnant mouse whom he had injected with a mock influenza. This reacted with her immune system to give her a constant, feverish temperature. The mice were confirmed to have many of the same behaviors autistic humans display such as a lack of socialization and a repeated pattern of behaviors. The doctor noted that these mice also had leaky intestines, which is not a surprise, as 40-90% of autistic people suffer problems of the gastrointestinal variety. To repair the intestinal problem, Patterson introduced a microbe to their GI tract. Interestingly, when the intestines healed and no longer leaked, those same autistic traits decreased as well. Much like the endocrine and GI connection, intestinal health and mental health are linked directly, and both contribute to the health of the other.

Recent studies on the connection between autism and inflammation backed these findings as people researched autism spectrum disorders, or ASDs, and their connection to inflammation. How autism is developed isn't completely known. However, inflammation in the womb, such as when a mother has a constant fever as seen in Patterson's mouse study, can certainly be one of the causes. During one study, it was found that these children often display many similar inflammation patterns as those with autoimmune diseases. Research is still being done to see if brain inflammation is linked to the high seizure risk in those with autism, as it is one of the theories on the matter. If the full connections between chronic inflammation and autism in humans are understood, then, eventually, it could be cured. As the mice study shows, it is often linked to the GI tract and a shortage of vital gut microbes. However, mice and humans are different organisms, and although the findings are an excellent start, it is just that. The key to eliminating autism in infants could very well be within the GI tract.

Autism is a mental condition that affects social behavior, mood, and judgment. An autistic person will have difficulty forming relationships and will often isolate themselves or be antisocial. They have a very difficult time understanding abstract or complicated concepts such as make-believe. A child with autism who has a young sibling might get angry if that sibling proclaims he has superpowers. People without autism might agree with this younger child and encourage their imagination in some way, like offering a blanket as a cape or calling them by their superhero name. However, because his proclamation isn't factual, the child with autism won't understand the reasoning behind it. How violent the response is, depends on other factors and can range from yelling to physical violence depending on each case. Fortunately, once this child is taught right from wrong, they will not stray from the guidelines. Strict rules and simple ways of following them is often how the brain of an autistic person operates, as judgment and grey areas are a very complicated and abstract concept.

The studies involving the connection between mental health and intestinal health are still quite new and underdeveloped. However, the current research greatly suggests that the key to understanding mental health and helping to alleviate depression and anxiety is to start with what is in the stomach. Though no drug exists thus far, staying informed about how lifestyle can contribute to the health of the GI tract is the first step toward your best physical and mental health. The research backs up the theory of how the anti-inflammation diet can benefit several aspects of life. Though some things are thus far incurable, such as Crohn's disease, autoimmune diseases, autism and many other inflammation-induced health complications, the anti-inflammation diet can help to manage the inflammation that can create uncomfortable symptoms. Changing to, and sticking with, the anti-inflammation diet, as well as, increasing physical activity in your daily routine can set in motion a series of events within your body. Doing so will heal your endocrine system, raise productivity levels, create a healthy immune system, which will decrease illness and infection, elevate the mood and work to clear depression and anxiety from the mind. Regardless of a person's lifestyle, the anti-inflammation diet benefits everyone in every way a diet can.

Why is this all important information? That is because knowing how the body is all interwoven as a single unit and not a single symptom can help you understand just how important it is to take care of it and provide it with what it needs. The body is a remarkable machine. But it can't operate as it's designed to without the proper components, and these components are found in the anti-inflammation diet. Things to remember when it comes to the anti-inflammation diet. There are no drawbacks. Only benefits. Unlike the medical anti-inflammatory drugs that can cause their own sets of health concerns, the diet only benefits the body in every aspect. It is always important to know the ingredients in foods that come from a grocery store, and whole foods are always the best option if it is unclear if something is healthy or not. Remembering to mix it up once in a while is important too, as different nutrients and benefits come from different foods, and eating the same thing every day can become boring and unsatisfying. Adding an exercise program to the anti-inflammation diet is not only essential to remain strong, flexible and, coordinated, it can also count as an anti-inflammatory and anti-depression treatment method on its own. And although it may not cure everything, this diet will help alleviate symptoms of chronic inflammation-induced diseases and complications such as rheumatoid arthritis, fibromyalgia, and Crohn's disease. Few things it can cure, however, are metabolic syndrome, obesity, and high blood pressure. As mental health goes, it is a very strong factor into whether a person has persistent depression and anxiety, as the intestines and mental health are two sides of the same coin. Above all, it is most important to remember that a healthy lifestyle added to the anti-inflammation diet will benefit your health, your mind, and your life.

Conclusion

Thanks for making it through to the end of *Healthy Brain, Healthy Gut, Healthy Life: How Anti-Inflammatory Diet Can Relieve Stress and Anxiety*, let's hope it was informative and able to provide you with all of the tools you need to achieve your physical and mental health goals.

The next step is to remember the knowledge this book has offered and put it into practice in your everyday life. Remember to be mindful of the long and short-term effects that unhealthy foods have on the body and mental status. When choosing what to eat, remember the listed foods in the anti-inflammation diet, and to experiment with combinations of flavors and textures. Finally, always keep in mind that the stomach can be the root cause of many seemingly unrelated health problems and that changing diet and lifestyle can help to decrease the risk of cancer, heart disease, autoimmune diseases, depression, anxiety, and diabetes. It is also important to keep in mind that, thought this diet may not cure some diseases such as the autoimmune diseases or fibromyalgia, it can alleviate the symptoms and help to make coping with these diseases easier for a person who lived with them. It is important to remember to always balance antibiotics with probiotics and why those probiotics are essential to a healthy brain and body. Always do your best to provide the body with what it needs. If it has everything it needs such as vitamins, nutrients, healthy fats, complex carbohydrates, and protein, it will function at its best so that you can be at your best. Remember that the key is to benefit the whole body, and live a happy, healthy life! Hopefully, you found this book helpful, and that you'll take the information with you on your road to a healthier, happier you.

Healthy Brain, Healthy Gut, Healthy Life

Finally, if you found this book useful in any way, a review on Amazon is always appreciated!

31909854R00033

Made in the USA
Middletown, DE
03 January 2019